Management of MDR-TB: A field guide

A companion document to *Guidelines for the programmatic management of drug-resistant tuberculosis*

WHO Library Cataloguing-in-Publication Data:

Management of MDR-TB : a field guide : a companion document to guidelines for programmatic management of drug-resistant tuberculosis : integrated management of adolescent and adult illness (IMAI).

"WHO/HTM/TB/2008.402a".

1.Tuberculosis, Multidrug-resistant – drug therapy. 2.Tuberculosis, Multidrug- resistant – prevention and control. 3.Antitubercular agents – administration and dosage. 4.Directly observed therapy - methods. 5.Delivery of health care, Integrated - organization and administration. 6.Antiretroviral therapy, Highly active. 7.Chronic disease - therapy 8.Practice guidelines. I.Partners in Health (Organization) II.World Health Organization.

ISBN 978 92 4 154776 5 (NLM classification: WF 310)

Printed in Italy

Acknowledgements

WHO gratefully acknowledges the contributions of Kwonjune Seung and Hind Satti, the authors of this module. In creating this module, they drew upon the experience of Partners In Health (PIH), an international health NGO with over 20 years of experience in the treatment of HIV and MDR-TB in resource-limited settings.

Integrated Management of Adolescent and Adult Illness (IMAI) is a multi-departmental project at WHO that produces guidelines and training materials for first-level health facility workers in low-resource settings. The WHO IMAI team collaborated closely for several months with Drs. Seung and Satti on the content and structure of this module. No experts involved declared a conflict of interest.

Foreword

Multidrug-resistant tuberculosis (MDR-TB) and extensively drug-resistant tuberculosis (XDR-TB) increasingly occur in resource-constrained settings. In the context of a national response to MDR- and XDR-TB, health workers in TB clinics (in district hospitals and some accredited health centres) will need to diagnose MDR-TB, initiate second-line anti-TB drugs, and monitor MDR-TB treatment.

Management of MDR-TB: a field guide was created to help health workers carry out these tasks. It is a job aid that medical officers and TB nurses are meant use frequently during the day for quick reference. This module is closely related to other clinical guideline modules in the Integrated Management of Adolescent and Adult Illness (IMAI) series. In particular, the approach to chronic disease management is taken from ***General principles of good chronic care*** in the IMAI series.

It is based on the Emergency Update 2008 of ***Guidelines for programmatic management of drug-resistant tuberculosis*** (WHO/HTM/TB/2008.402), and may be considered a companion document to these guidelines. It also draws on the experience of the international health NGO Partners In Health (PIH) in many countries, and the Lesotho version of this module that was adapted by the Lesotho National TB Programme. This module should be introduced to health workers in the context of a training course with a strong emphasis on TB-HIV co-management.

This document is expected to remain valid until 2010 when a fully revised second edition of the ***Guidelines for programmatic management of drug-resistant tuberculosis*** will be published. The Stop TB Department at WHO Headquarters in Geneva will be responsible for initiating a review of this document at that time.

For more information about IMAI, please see http://www.who.int/hiv/capacity/ or contact imaimail@who.int. For more information about global TB/HIV initiatives, see http://www.stoptb.org/wg/tb_hiv/ or http://www.who.int/tb/hiv/en/.

WHO HIV/AIDS Department—IMAI Project

WHO Stop TB Department—TB/HIV and Drug Resistance Unit

Chronic Care for MDR-TB cross-references other IMAI/IMCI guideline modules for primary health care. These include:

- ***Acute care***: management of common acute problems that arise during chronic care.
- ***Palliative care***: for management of pain and issues related to end-of-life care. Page numbers beginning with "P" refer to this guideline module.
- ***Chronic HIV care with ART and prevention***: for management of HIV and antiretroviral therapy.

Use the general principles of good chronic care

See IMAI module with this title for more detail.

1. Develop a treatment partnership with your patient.
2. Focus on your patient's concerns and priorities.
3. Use the 5 As—Assess, Advise, Agree, Assist, Arrange.
4. Support the patient education and self-management.
5. Organize proactive follow-up.
6. Involve "expert patients", peer educators and support staff at your health facility. (These are referred to in these guidelines as lay providers).
7. Link the patient to community-based resources and support.
8. Use written information—registers, treatment plans, the patient calendars, treatment cards—to document, monitor, and remind.
9. Work as a clinical team (and hold team meetings).
10. Assure continuity of care.

TABLE OF CONTENTS

ROLES AND RELATIONSHIPS

Specialized MDR-TB inpatient ward

- MDR-TB inpatient ward for sick, complicated, or XDR-TB patients;
- Training centre: attachments for district hospital and health centre staff;
- 24-hour hotline for district hospital clinical teams on MDR-TB management;
- Mentoring and supervision of district hospital clinical teams;
- Central pharmacy for second-line anti-TB drugs; provide supplies of drugs to district hospital pharmacies for each MDR-TB patient in treatment.

Outpatient clinic (district hospital and accredited health centres)

- Diagnose and treat uncomplicated MDR-TB patients;
- Receive down-referral of stable patients from inpatient ward;
- Regular consultations and laboratory monitoring of MDR-TB patients;
- Maintain MDR-TB register and copies of MDR-TB treatment cards for all patients;
- Nurses refer to district medical officer for design of individualized regimens or management of complicated cases;
- Request drugs for the patients and use feedback form for central pharmacy;
- Select treatment supporter after discussion with the patient and health centre;
- Provide training and supervision to MDR-TB treatment supporters;
- Provide incentives and transportation support to the patient and treatment supporter.

Health centre

- Provide injections (in some cases).
- Manage minor side-effects that do not require referral to district hospital.
- Follow-up of MDR-TB contacts.

The patient

- Hold monthly box of drugs.
- Take doses under supervision of MDR-TB treatment supporter.
- Attend monthly consultations at district hospital with treatment supporter.
- Provide sputum to treatment supporter on monthly basis.

MDR-TB treatment supporter

- Supervise both doses (morning and evening), including injections at the health centre.
- Provide injections (in some cases).
- Accompany the patient to all medical consultations.
- Provide sputum bottles to the patient on monthly basis for sputum collection.
- Record doses on Category 4 treatment card.
- Take injectable drugs and supplies to health centre every month; return box to district hospital at end of month.
- Screen the patient's family for HIV and TB.

Sequence of care for MDR-TB

2 Education and support

- Explain treatment, follow-up care.
- Assess and support adherence to anti-TB and ARV therapy.
- Assess quality of DOT by treatment supporter.
- For HIV-positive the patients, give post-test, ongoing support.

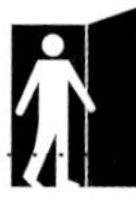

1 Triage

- The patient and treatment supporter return for follow-up.
- Retrieve facility records.

The patient continues with treatment support and directly observed therapy.

Family and friends, peer support, community health workers.

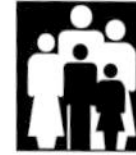

8 Arrange

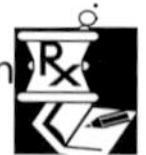

- Dispense and record medication.
- Schedule follow-up; order labs.
- Link with community services.
- Record data on Category 4 treatment card.
- Provide incentives to the patient and treatment supporter.

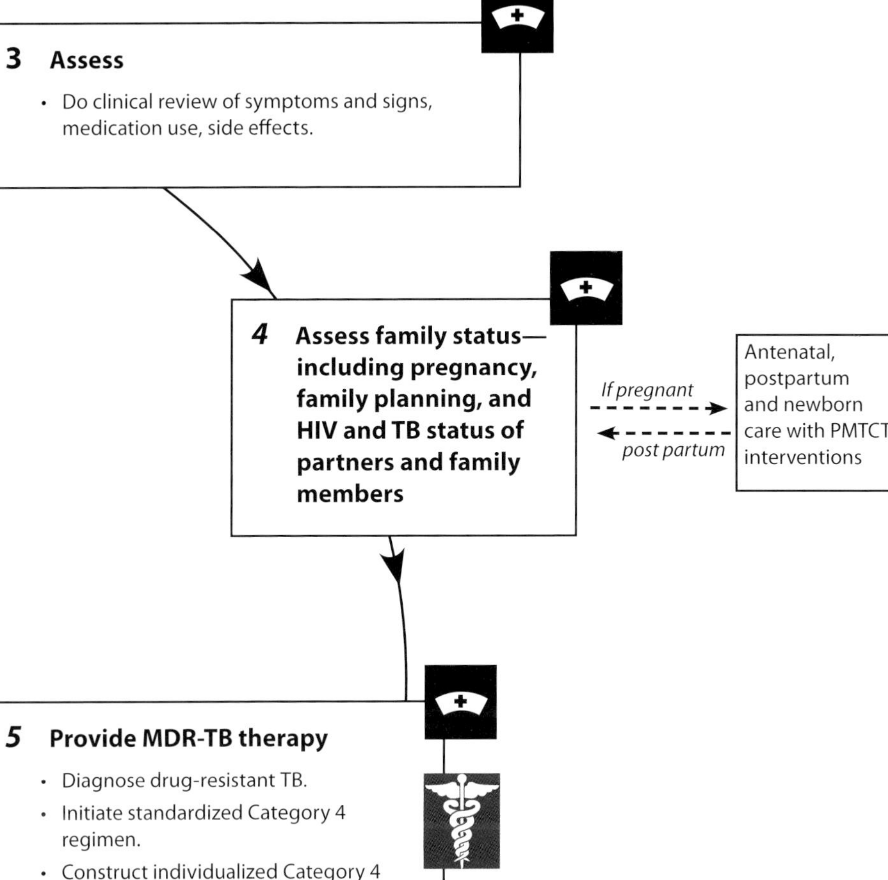
3 Assess
• Do clinical review of symptoms and signs, medication use, side effects.
4 Assess family status—including pregnancy, family planning, and HIV and TB status of partners and family members
If pregnant
post partum
Antenatal, postpartum and newborn care with PMTCT interventions
5 Provide MDR-TB therapy
• Diagnose drug-resistant TB.
• Initiate standardized Category 4 regimen.
• Construct individualized Category 4 regimen according to DST results.
6 If HIV-positive, provide chronic HIV care
• Use IMAI chronic HIV care.
7 Manage common problems
• Acute illness (use IMAI Acute care)
• Side effects
• Chronic problems.
Consult with specialists (HIV, TB or thoracic surgery).

1 Triage

- Greet the patient and treatment supporter.
- If this is a follow-up the patient, retrieve the records.
- Weigh the patient and record the weight on the MDR-TB treatment card.
- Give tissues to smear-positive patients and instruct them to cover their mouths and noses when they cough. No-touch receptacles for disposal of used tissues should be available in the waiting areas.
- All TB patients should wait in a well-ventilated area. New or suspected MDR-TB cases or smear-positive cases should be seen before smear-negative patients.
- Smear-positive MDR-TB patients co-infected with HIV should not be seen in the HIV/ART area.

2 Educate and support the patient on each visit

2.1 Directly observed treatment

- Agree on a time and place to meet the patient. Do not make the patient wait.
- Check the drugs to be sure that they are correct. Watch the patient swallow all the drugs.
- Record on the treatment card each time the patient takes the drugs.
- Be aware of possible side-effects. Have the patient eat food with the tablets if needed to reduce nausea. Refer the patient to the health facility if the side-effects continue.
- Encourage the patient to continue coming for treatment.
- Respond quickly if the patient misses a scheduled treatment. When the patient misses a dose for more than 24 hours, visit their home. Find out what caused the interruption. Give the treatment. If you are unable to find the patient or convince them to continue the treatment, contact the health facility for help without delay.
- Accompany the patient to the health facility each month. Show the patient's treatment card. Review how they is doing and discuss any problems.
- Make arrangements if you or the patient will be away for a few days. Give the patient enough drugs to self-administer for a maximum of one week or refer them to the health facility to decide what is to be done. Someone else may be asked to help during this time.
- Give the patient sputum bottles every month and coach them on how to produce a good sputum sample. Take the sputum with you to the monthly appointment at the facility.

2.2 MDR-TB treatment supporters

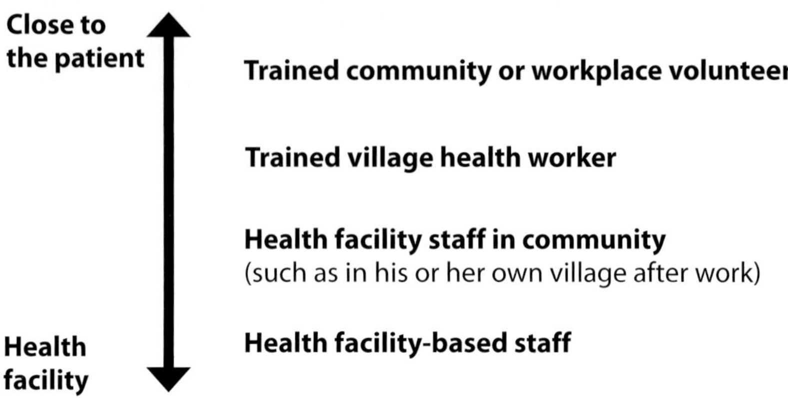

The treatment supporter should be someone who:

- ✓ is chosen by or is acceptable to the patient;
- ✓ is committed to support the patient for a long time;
- ✓ has received MDR-TB specific training;
- ✓ is available to observe doses twice a day;
- ✓ is available to accompany patients to clinic and lab appointments;
- ✓ provides support to fewer than two MDR-TB patients;
- ✓ should not be immunosuppressed.

2.3 Adherence support

❖ First visit (diagnosis):

- Prepare the patient (see 2.4, *Adherence preparation*).
- Provide list of possible treatment supporters (the village health worker, a health facilty or other community member), and decide on a treatment supporter.
- Give food package and transportation money to the patient.

❖ In between first and second visit:

- Contact health centre; arrange for injections to be given daily for at least six months.

❖ Second visit (first day of treatment):

- Treatment supporter comes for the first time with the patient.
- If treatment supporter has not been trained in MDR-TB, provide standard training for MDR-TB treatment supporters.
- Assess understanding of doses (use *Dosing Job Aid*).
- Give Category 4 drugs (one month supply box) to the patient.
- Give one month supply box of injectable and related supplies to treatment supporter (to take to health centre).
- Give *Category 4 treatment card*, exercise book, and pen to the treatment supporter.
- Give sputum bottles for next month.
- Give food package and transportation money to the patient.
- Give transportation money to the treatment supporter.

❖ Follow-up visits (monthly):

- Treatment supporter must accompany the patient to all follow-up visits.
- Assess the patient is and the treatment supporter is understanding of doses (use *Dosing Job Aid*). Check that the patient's morning and evening regimen is correct in the treatment supporter's exercise book. Check for side-effects.
- Update the facility-held *Category 4 treatment card*.
- Verify that the patient is being supervised correctly by the treatment supporter.
- Give sputum bottles for the next month.
- Give the food package and transportation money to the patient.
- Give transportation money and incentive to the treatment supporter if he/she has fulfilled his/her monthly responsibilities.

2.4 Adherence preparation

Prepare for MDR-TB therapy:

ASSESS

- The patient's understanding of anti-TB drug resistance, and how he/she was infected with a drug-resistant strain;
- His/her understanding of MDR-TB therapy;
- Whether the patient has demonstrated an ability to keep appointments, and to adhere to other medications;
- Whether the patient knows his/her HIV serostatus.

ADVISE

- Drug-resistant TB:
  - is created when TB patients do not take anti-TB drugs regularly;
  - can be transmitted to family and friends;
  - can be easily transmitted to people living with HIV.
- Offer HIV testing if the patient does not know their serostatus.
- MDR-TB treatment lasts for at least 2 years.
- Second-line anti-TB drugs are weaker than first-line anti-TB drugs. Every single dose must be taken at the correct time of the day. If not, there is a good chance treatment may fail.
- There is no other treatment for MDR-TB.
- Second-line anti-TB drugs have many side-effects, but these can be managed. The clinical team must communicate closely with the MDR-TB treatment supporter about side-effects.
- The patient is most infectious during the first few months when he/she is still smear positive. Windows and doors should be left open in the home to increase ventilation.

AGREE

- that the patient is willing to undergo at least 2 years of treatment with second-line anti-TB drugs;
- that the patient is willing to receive directly observed therapy;
- On who will observe the therapy? community health worker at home or a health worker at a nearby facility?
- that the patient understands the programme will stop treatment if he/she does not take doses regularly;
- that the patient is willing to come monthly to the MDR-TB clinic for follow-up (usually at a district hospital).

ASSIST

- by discussing how taking medications can be integrated into work and home routines;
- by giving food packages if needed;
- by giving support for transportation. If the patient lives in a remote area, discuss options such the patient moving closer to the clinic for a period of time;
- by referring the patient to an MDR-TB therapeutic support group.

ARRANGE

- for injections to be given at the health centre nearest to the patient's home;
- to educate the treatment supporter about MDR-TB and how to observe MDR-TB therapy.

2.5 Adherence monitoring

Monitor and support adherence:

ASSESS

- Check the patient's understanding of the information given previously—make sure the patient understands the illness, treatment and possible side effects.
- Review the medications (use *Dosing Job Aid*). Make sure the patient is taking the correct dose.
- Determine whether there is an adherence problem.
- Ask questions in a respectful and non-judgmental way. Pose the questions in a manner that makes it easier for the patients to be truthful:
  - "Many patients have trouble taking their medications. What trouble do you have?"
  - "Can you tell me when and how you take each pill?"
  - "When is it most difficult for you to take the pills?"
- If there is poor adherence, determine the nature of the problem:
  - Side-effects?
  - Forgot?
  - Problems with the treatment supporter?
  - Financial or transport problems?
  - Not enough food?
  - Work problems?
  - Seldom at home and disorganized?
  - Another medical problem?
  - Alcohol abuse?
  - Depression?

ADVISE

- Reinforce the information given previously, and why adherence is important.
- Explain which drugs are likely causing the side effects.
- Suggest home remedies that could help with side effects (see *Palliative Care*): symptom management and end-of-life care

AGREE

- Agree on any changes to the treatment regimen and solutions to adherence problems (if these are occuring).

ASSIST

- Be empathetic and supportive.
- Refer the patient for food packages, or economic support if needed.
- Make sure that the patient has aids or skills that could improve their adherence (e.g. how to use a diary).
- Make sure the patient has adherence support:
  - Obtain help from family and friends.
  - Discuss problems with the treatment supporter to find solutions.
- Carry out a home visit if adherence is a problem.
- Refer the patient to an MDR-TB therapeutic support group if depression or anxiety is a problem.

ARRANGE

- Fill out the MDR-TB treatment card.
- Set the date of next clinic visit. Set the date of home visit if necessary.
- Make sure that the patient and treatment supporter understand the follow-up plan and how to contact the clinic team if there is a problem.

2.6 Education

As needed, remind the patient of one or more relevant messages (on right):

The patient	Advice
If the patient has not yet brought household contacts for examination or testing	All household members with cough should be tested
If the patient is unfamiliar with the drugs, or a change occurs in the regimen	Describe the type, colour, and amount of drugs to be taken. Describe how often drugs should be taken and for how long
If the patient feels better	*"Even after you feel better, you must continue taking drugs for the entire treatment period"*
If the patient is planning to travel or move	*"If you plan to travel or move from the area, please inform me. We can make arrangements so that you will not miss any treatments"*
If the patient has missed a dose	*"To be cured, you must take all of the recommended drugs together, for the entire time. If you do not take all of the drugs, you will continue to spread TB to others"*
If the patient complains about continuing treatment	*"Taking only some of the drugs, or taking them irregularly, is dangerous and can make the disease impossible to cure"*

If it is time for a follow-up sputum examination:

Advisor	Message
Explain the need for the sputum examination	*"TB germs cannot be seen with the eye. A laboratory technician must examine sputum under a microscope to see if there are still TB germs and if you are getting better"*
Explain the need for the sputum culture	*"The laboratory technician will try to grow TB germs from your sputum. If no TB germs grow, this means that your lungs are becoming very clear of TB"*
Review: Ask verification questions (to ensure that the patient remembers important messages and knows what to do next). Reinforce earlier messages or give more information as needed	

3 Assess: Clinical review of symptoms and signs, medication use, side-effects, complications

3.1 Ask	3.2 Look
If this is first visit: • Review the patient's past medical history, including their past history of TB treatments. **For all visits:** • How have you been? • Have you needed urgent medical care? If yes, ask for record/diagnosis. • Have your TB symptoms improved? – Cough? Sputum? – Difficult breathing? – Fever/night sweats? – Weight loss? • Have you had any side-effects? – Nausea/vomiting? – Fatigue? – Skin rash? – Tingling in hands or feet? – Deafness? Ringing of ears? – Headache? – Seizures? Loss of consciousness? – Feeling anxious? Feeling sad or unhappy? • What problems have you had taking the medicines? Have you missed any doses? • Have you had any problems with your treatment supporter? • What else do you want to talk about?	**In all patients:** • Weigh the patient. Calculate weight gain or loss. Record. If weight loss, ask about food intake • Measure temperature • Count respiratory rate • Look for pallor. If pallor, check haemoglobin • Look at whites of the eye—yellow? • Look for thrush **If any new symptoms:** • Do further assessment of symptoms. (See IMAI *Acute care*)

3.3 Lab and clinical follow-up

At baseline, before starting Category 4 regimen:

- Check complete blood count (CBC), Aspartate Transaminase (AST), Alanaine Transaminase (ALT), bilirubin, creatinine, potassium.
- For women, do a pregnancy test.

<table>
<tr><th>Month</th><th>Clinical consult</th><th>Smear</th><th>Culture</th><th>DST</th><th>AST, ALT, bili†</th><th>Cr, K†</th><th>TSH</th></tr>
<tr><td>1</td><td rowspan="3">Every 2 weeks</td><td>√</td><td></td><td></td><td>√</td><td>√</td><td></td></tr>
<tr><td>2</td><td>√</td><td></td><td></td><td>√</td><td>√</td><td>√*</td></tr>
<tr><td>3</td><td>√</td><td>√</td><td></td><td>√</td><td>√</td><td></td></tr>
<tr><td>4</td><td rowspan="10">Monthly</td><td>√</td><td></td><td></td><td></td><td></td><td></td></tr>
<tr><td>5</td><td>√</td><td></td><td></td><td></td><td></td><td></td></tr>
<tr><td>6</td><td>√</td><td>√</td><td>√</td><td></td><td></td><td>√</td></tr>
<tr><td>7</td><td>√</td><td></td><td></td><td></td><td></td><td></td></tr>
<tr><td>8</td><td>√</td><td></td><td></td><td></td><td></td><td></td></tr>
<tr><td>9</td><td>√</td><td>√</td><td></td><td></td><td></td><td></td></tr>
<tr><td>10</td><td>√</td><td></td><td></td><td></td><td></td><td></td></tr>
<tr><td>11</td><td>√</td><td></td><td></td><td></td><td></td><td></td></tr>
<tr><td>12</td><td>√</td><td>√</td><td>√</td><td></td><td></td><td>√</td></tr>
<tr><td>until completion</td><td>Monthly</td><td>Every three months</td><td>Every six months</td><td></td><td></td><td></td></tr>
</table>

† Liver function and renal function tests may be done at any time when clinically indicated.

*** TSH in month two is recommended in settings with early onset of hypothyroidism.**

For patients co-infected with HIV:

- Check the patient's haemoglobin before starting AZT and at four, eight and 12 weeks of treatment, or if there are any clinical symptoms or signs of anaemia.
- Check the patient's CD4 at baseline and then every six months.

4 Assess family status—pregnancy, family planning, HIV and TB status of partners and family members

All women of childbearing age should be using a reliable contraceptive method.

- If a patient's pregnancy status is uncertain, perform a pregnancy test.
- Give reproductive choice and family planning counselling. See Annex A.4.
- Injectable contraceptives are preferred.
- If a patient is HIV-positive, her partner should also use condoms.

If patient is HIV-positive, facilitate HIV testing of partner(s) and children.

All household contacts should be screened for TB.

- A household contact is a person who lives (that is, sleeps and eats at least one meal per day) in the home of a TB patient and is therefore at greater risk of being infected.
- Ask about symptoms of TB: cough, night sweats, etc.
    - For household contacts with symptoms: perform smear, culture, drug susceptibility testing (DST), and a chest X-ray.
    - For household contacts without symptoms: perform a chest X-ray.
- Keep all chest X-rays on file for future reference.

5 Provide MDR-TB therapy

5.1 Treatment categories

<table>
<tr><th>Disease Site</th><th>Laboratory results</th><th colspan="2">Type of Patient</th><th>Recommended treatment category</th></tr>
<tr><td rowspan="6">Pulmonary</td><td rowspan="5">Sputum smear-positive</td><td colspan="2">New</td><td>CAT 1</td></tr>
<tr><td rowspan="4">Previously treated</td><td>Relapse</td><td>CAT 2</td></tr>
<tr><td>Treatment after default</td><td>CAT 2</td></tr>
<tr><td>Treatment after failure</td><td>CAT 4</td></tr>
<tr><td>Chronic or MDR-TB</td><td>CAT 4</td></tr>
<tr><td>Sputum smear-negative†</td><td colspan="2"></td><td>CAT 1</td></tr>
<tr><td>Extrapulmonary†</td><td colspan="3"></td><td>CAT 1</td></tr>
</table>

† Pulmonary sputum smear-negative cases and extrapulmonary cases may occasionally fit the definition of "previously treated" (relapse, treatment after default, treatment after failure, or chronic cases). Diagnosis should be based on bacteriological and pathological evidence.

5.2 Start empiric regimen in patients at risk of drug resistance

Medium Risk

Migrant worker with new TB	Send two sputums for culture and DST. Start Category 1 regimen.
Health worker with new TB	Send two sputums for culture and DST. Start Category 1 regimen.
Treatment after relapse or default	Send two sputums for culture and DST. Start Category 2 regimen.

High Risk

Household contact of known MDR-TB patient with new TB	Send two sputums for culture and DST. Start individualized Category 4 regimen based on DST of contact.
Probable treatment failure: • Smear-positive in fifth month of Category 1 or 2 • HIV-positive and clinically worsening during Category 1 or 2	Send two sputums for culture and DST. Start standardized Category 4 regimen. There are many reasons for clinical worsening in HIV-positive patients besides treatment failure. Consult a specialist for advice.
History of treatment with second-line drugs	Send two sputums for culture and DST. Will need an individualized Category 4 regimen. Consult a specialist for advice.

5.3 Summary of steps to initiate MDR-TB therapy

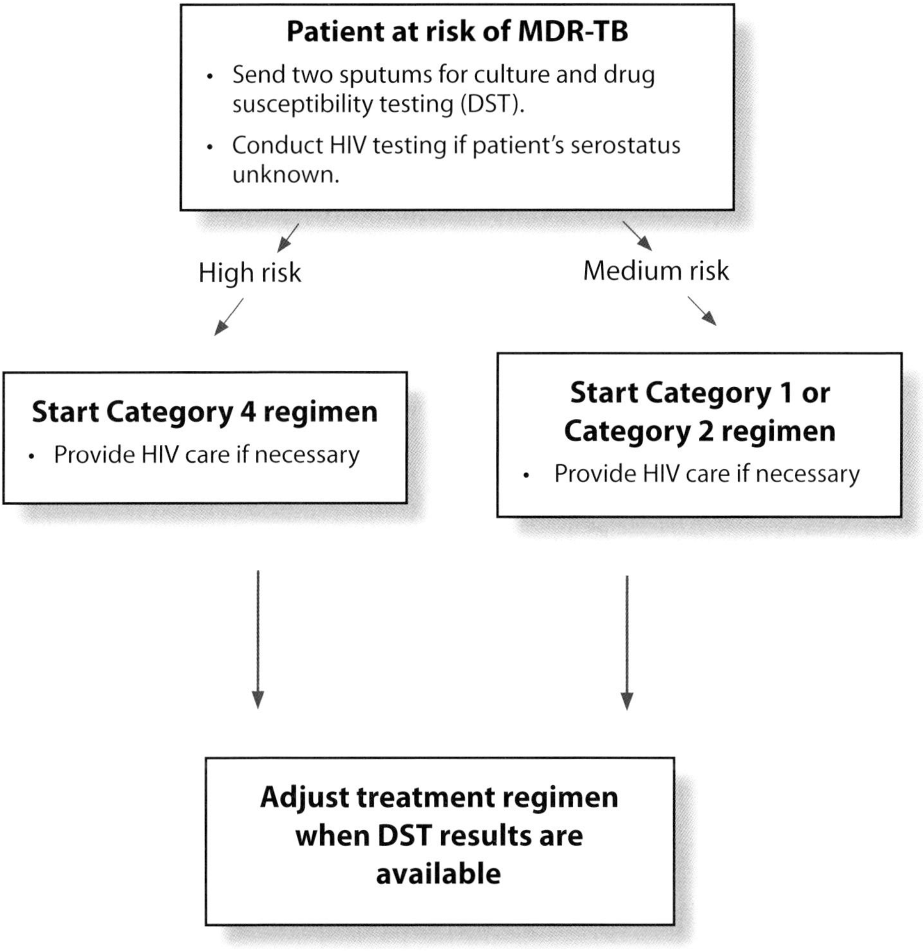

Patient at risk of MDR-TB

- Send two sputums for culture and drug susceptibility testing (DST).
- Conduct HIV testing if patient's serostatus unknown.

High risk → **Start Category 4 regimen**

- Provide HIV care if necessary

Medium risk → **Start Category 1 or Category 2 regimen**

- Provide HIV care if necessary

→ **Adjust treatment regimen when DST results are available**

5.4 Standardized Category 4 regimen

Standardized Category 4 regimen[†]:

Z - Km - Lfx - Eto - Cs - PAS

Criteria for patient to be started on a standardized Category 4 regimen

1. Is patient pregnant?
2. Is there jaundice or a known liver problem?
3. Is there chronic illness such as diabetes mellitus, heart or kidney disease, etc.?
4. Is the patient a household contact of a patient with MDR-TB?
5. Has the patient ever taken second-line anti-TB drugs?

NO to all

Give the standardized Category 4 regimen.

YES to any question

Do not start the standardized Category 4 regimen. The patient will need individualized Category 4 regimen—consult, or refer to a MDR-TB specialist.

[†] All patients receiving cycloserine or terizidone should receive pyridoxine. The recommended daily dose is 50 mg for every 250 mg of cycloserine.

Treatment phases

	Duration	Characteristics
Initial phase	At least six months and until sputum smears and cultures are continuously negative	• Close monitoring for side-effects • At least five drugs • Includes injectable
Continuation phase	12-18 months	• Fewer side-effects • Usually only oral drugs

Duration of injectable

- ❖ The decision to stop the injectable should depend on the clinical status of the patient, the bacteriological data (smears and cultures), the chest X-ray, and the DST results.
- ❖ In patients infected with highly resistant strains, the clinician may opt to continue the injectable during the entire course of treatment. In these cases, the clinician may decrease the frequency to three times per week.

5.5 Adjust the Category 4 regimen according to drug susceptibility testing (DST) results

General principles

1. Include at least five drugs.
2. Include any first-line drugs to which the strain is susceptible.
3. Include an injectable for a prolonged period.
4. Include a quinolone.
5. Consider drug resistance data (of individual or region) and the patient's treatment history when designing a regimen.

First-line	**Second-line**			
	Injectable	**Quinolone**	**Other 2nd line**	**Other drugs**
Isoniazid	Streptomycin	Ofloxacin	Ethionamide	[unclear efficacy]
Rifampicin	Kanamycin	Levofloxacin	Cycloserine	
Ethambutol	Capreomycin	Moxifloxacin	PAS	
Pyrazinamide				

Resistance pattern	Change to
Pan-susceptible	Category 1 (HREZ)
H (+/- S)	R - E- Z (six to nine months)
Polyresistant but not MDR	Continue the empiric second-line regimen. Consult with specialist. Patient may require a combination of first and second-line drugs.
HR HRE	Z - S - Lfx - Eto - Cs - PAS
HREZ	S - Lfx - Eto - Cs - PAS
HRS HRES HREZS	Km - Lfx - Eto - Cs - PAS
Resistance to any second-line drug	Continue the empiric second-line regimen. Consult with a specialist.

❖ Patients who have failed first-line TB treatment regimens, such as Category 1 or Category 2, should be started on Category 4 unless there is clear evidence of non-adherence. There are a number of polyresistant DST patterns that are not likely to occur after failures of first-line TB regimens, and are probably laboratory errors.

5.6 Anti-TB drug dosing

Adults and adolescents

Drug	Weight class			
	Average daily dosage	**33-50 KG**	**51–70 KG**	**>70 KG (max dose)**
Isoniazid (H) (100, 300 mg)	4–6 mg/kg daily	200-300 mg	300 mg	300 mg
Rifampicin (R) (150, 300 mg)	10–20 mg/kg daily	450-600 mg	600 mg	600 mg
Ethambutol (E) (400 mg)	25 mg/kg daily	800-1200 mg	1200-1600 mg	1600-2000 mg
Pyrazinamide (Z) (500 mg)	30–40 mg/kg daily	1000-1750 mg	1750 mg	2000-2500 mg
Streptomycin (S) (1 g vial)	15–20 mg/kg daily	500-750 mg	1000 mg	1000 mg
Kanamycin (Km) (1 g vial)	15–20 mg/kg daily	500-750 mg	1000 mg	1000 mg
Capreomycin (Cm) (1 g vial)	15–20 mg/kg daily	500-750 mg	1000 mg	1000 mg
Ofloxacin (Ofx) (200 mg)	Usual adult dose is 800 mg	800 mg	800 mg	800-1000 mg
Levofloxacin (Lfx) (250 mg, 500 mg)	Usual adult dose is 1000 mg	750 mg	750-1000 mg	750-1000 mg
Moxifloxacin (Mfx) (400 mg)	Usual adult dose is 400 mg	400 mg	400 mg	400 mg
Ethionamide (Eto) (250 mg)	15–20 mg/kg daily	500 mg	750 mg	750–1000 mg
Cycloserine (Cs) (250 mg)	15–20 mg/kg daily	500 mg	750 mg	750–1000 mg
Terizidone (Trd) (250 mg)	15–20 mg/kg daily	500 mg	750 mg	750–1000 mg
PASER® (4 g sachets)	150 mg/kg daily	8 g	8 g	8 -12 g

Children

Medication (common presentation)	Dose	Maximum daily dose
Isoniazid (H)	4–6 mg/kg daily or 8–12 mg 3 x wk	300 mg
Rifampicin (R)	10–20 mg/kg daily	600 mg
Ethambutol (E)	25 mg/kg daily	1200 mg
Pyrazinamide (Z)	30–40 mg/kg daily	1500 mg
Streptomycin (S)	20–40 mg/kg daily	1000 mg
Kanamycin (Km)	15–30 mg/kg daily	1000 mg
Capreomycin (Cm)	15–30 mg/kg daily	1000 mg
Ofloxacin (Ofx)	15–20 mg/kg daily	800 mg
Levofloxacin (Lfx)	15–25 mg/kg daily	1000 mg
Moxifloxacin (Mfx)	7.5–10 mg/kg daily	400 mg
Ethionamide (Eto)	15–20 mg/kg daily	1000 mg
Cycloserine (Cs)	10–20 mg/kg daily	1000 mg
Terizidone (Trd)	10–20 mg/kg daily	1000 mg
Para-aminosalicylic acid (PAS)	150 mg/kg daily	8 g (PASER®)

❖ For all quinolones, the daily dose should be given in a single dose once a day.

❖ For ethionamide, cycloserine, and PAS, the daily dose is divided into morning and evening doses for better tolerance.

❖ All patients should receive pyridoxine. The recommended daily dose is 50 mg for every 250 mg of cycloserine/terizidone:

- 50 mg daily if they are receiving cycloserine 250 mg daily
- 100 mg daily if they are receiving cycloserine 500 mg daily
- 150 mg daily if they are receiving cycloserine 750 mg daily, etc.

5.7 Special considerations for pregnant women

- Pregnancy is not a contraindication to the treatment of MDR-TB.
- Discuss the risks and benefits with the mother.
- Start treatment of drug resistance in the second trimester, or sooner if the condition of the patient is severe. Since the majority of teratogenic effects occur in the first trimester, therapy may be delayed until the second trimester.
- Avoid injectable agents. For the most part, aminoglycosides should not be used in the regimens of pregnant patients and can be particularly toxic to the developing foetal ear. Capreomycin may carry the same risk of ototoxicity, but is the injectable drug of choice if an injectable agent cannot be avoided.
- Avoid ethionamide. Ethionamide can increase the risk of nausea and vomiting associated with pregnancy, and teratogenic effects have been observed in animal studies.

5.8 Special considerations for patients with renal insufficiency

Drug	Frequency	Recommended dose and frequency for patients with creatinine clearance < 30 ml/min, or for patients receiving haemodialysis
Isoniazid	No change	300 mg once daily, or 900 mg three times per week
Rifampicin	No change	600 mg once daily, or 600 mg three times per week
Ethambutol	Yes	15–25 mg/kg per dose three times per week (not daily)
Pyrazinamide	Yes	25–35 mg/kg per dose three times per week (not daily)
Ofloxacin	Yes	600–800 mg per dose three times per week (not daily)
Levofloxacin	Yes	750-1000 mg per dose three times per week (not daily)
Moxifloxacin	No change	400 mg once daily
Gatifloxacin	Yes	400 mg per dose three times per week (not daily)
Cycloserine	Yes	250 mg once daily, or 500 mg/dose three times per week
Terizidone	-	Recommendations not available
Ethionamide	No change	250–500 mg per dose daily
PAS	No change	4 g/dose, twice daily (PASER®)†
Streptomycin	Yes	12–15 mg/kg per dose two or three times per week (not daily)*
Kanamycin	Yes	12–15 mg/kg per dose two or three times per week (not daily)*
Capreomycin	Yes	12–15 mg/kg per dose two or three times per week (not daily)*

† Sodium salt formulations of PAS may result in an excessive sodium load and should be avoided in patients with renal insufficiency. Formulations of PAS that do not use the sodium salt can be used without the hazard of sodium retention.

* Caution should be used with the injectable agents in patients with renal function impairment because of the increased risk of both ototoxicity and nephrotoxicity.

5.9 Standardized Category 4 regimen instructions (for a 60 kg patient)

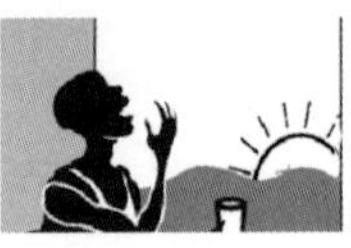

Pyrazinamide: 3½ tablets (1750 mg)

Kanamycin: 1 injection (1000 mg)

Levofloxacin: 2 tablets (500 mg)

Ethionamide: 1 tablet (250 mg)

Cycloserine: 1 capsule (250 mg)

PAS: 1 sachet (4 g)†

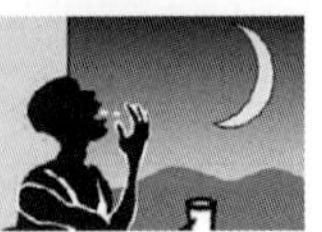

Ethionamide: 2 tablets (500 mg)

Cycloserine: 2 capsules (500 mg)

PAS: 1 sachet (4 g)†

Pyridoxine: 6 tablets (150 mg)

If on ART co-treatment:

AZT-3TC: 1 tablet

Cotrimoxazole: 1 tablet (960 mg)

If on ART co-treatment:

AZT-3TC: 1 tablet

EFZ: 1 tablet

If you have any of the following symptoms, report them to the health worker AT THE NEXT VISIT:

- Nausea or vomiting
- Diarrhoea
- Tingling, numb or painful feet or legs or hands.

SEEK CARE URGENTLY if you have:

- Skin rash
- Severe abdominal pain
- Yellow eyes
- Strange visions or thoughts
- Fatigue AND shortness of breath.

† PASER® formulation of PAS must be taken with an acidic liquid. See package insert for details.

5.10 Monitor Category 4 treatment outcome

- ❖ Signs of treatment failure:
  - Persistent or new weight loss
  - Persistent or new TB symptoms (fever, cough, sputum)
  - Persistently positive sputum smears or cultures
  - Smear or culture positive after being negative for some time.
- ❖ Other opportunistic infections can be easily confused with treatment failure. Call for advice.

6 Provide chronic HIV care

6.1 Cotrimoxazole (CTX) prophylaxis

All HIV-positive patients should be receiving cotrimoxazole prophylaxis.

Advise patients of the advantages of cotrimoxazole prophylaxis. Cotrimoxazole protects against Pneumocystis pneumonia (PCP), toxoplasmosis, bacterial infections, pneumonia and malaria.

Initiate

- Ask about previous history of sulpha allergy (to cotrimoxazole/Bactrim®/ Septrin®, S-P/Fansidar®)

Dispense a month's supply

- Give one double strength (960 mg) or two single-strength (480 mg) tablets daily.

Monitor

- Ask about symptoms. Check for rash and pallor.

Nausea	The patient should continue cotrimoxazole and take it with food. If there is severe or persistent vomiting, consult or refer.
Rash	If the patient has a generalized rash, a fixed drug reaction, peeling, or eye or mouth involvement, stop the cotrimoxazole and call for advice.
Pallor or haemoglobin < 8 g/dl or bleeding gums	Stop the cotrimoxazole. Call for advice or refer.
New jaundice	Stop the cotrimoxazole. Call for advice or refer.

6.2 Antiretroviral therapy (ART) co-treatment

- ART is not a reason to delay MDR-TB treatment!
- If the patient is not on ART, start ART co-treatment as soon as MDR-TB treatment is tolerated.
- The preferred ART regimen for patients on MDR-TB treatment is AZT-3TC-EFZ. However, if the patient is already taking ART, continue the same ART regimen.

How to start ART co-treatment in an MDR-TB patient (60 kg)

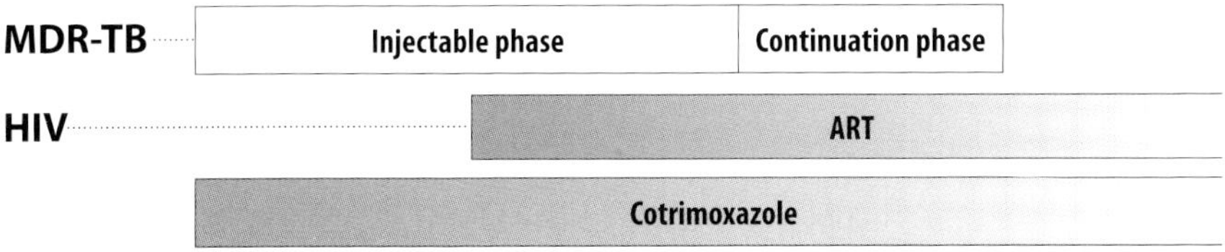

MDR-TB: Injectable phase | Continuation phase

HIV: ART

Cotrimoxazole

	TB initial phase-until tolerated	Until end of TB initial phase	During continuation phase	After TB treatment completed
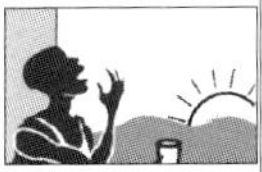	Z: Km: Lfx: Eto: Cs: PAS:	Z: Km: Lfx: Eto: Cs: PAS:	Z: Lfx: Eto: Cs: PAS:	
	CTX:	AZT-3TC: CTX:	AZT-3TC: CTX:	AZT-3TC: CTX:
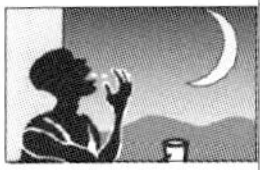	Eto: Cs: PAS: Pyridoxine:	Eto: Cs: PAS: Pyridoxine:	Eto: Cs: PAS: Pyridoxine:	
		AZT-3TC: EFZ:	AZT-3TC: EFZ:	AZT-3TC: EFZ:

6.3 Manage immune reconstitution syndrome

- Immune reconstitution syndrome (IRIS) is a syndrome that occurs when TB symptoms become worse in the first two to eight weeks of ART.
- IRIS is a sign that the immune system is starting to work again, and it does not mean that the ART is not working.
- If IRIS occurs, use non-steroidal anti-inflammatories such as ibuprofen.
- Corticosteroids can be used to suppress IRIS in severe cases. Give prednisone 0.5 mg/kg for up to 21 days. Do not stop ART without consulting with a specialist.

If ⟶ Then

Symptoms	How to manage
Worsening cough, increased sputum production	Consider other causes of cough, such as pneumonia. Send sputum for smear and culture If cough is moderate or severe, give prednisone
Worsening headache, new paralysis	If no history of meningitis, do full workup including lumbar puncture.
Enlarged lymph nodes	Continue TB therapy and ART
Abdominal distension	Give prednisone. Consult a specialist. Consider stopping ART if symptoms are severe

7 Manage common problems

7.1 Cough or difficult breathing

- Cough caused by TB may not improve for several months after the patient starts MDR-TB therapy.
- Patients may have worsening wheezing as lungs scar during the healing process.
- There may be a superimposed bronchitis or pneumonia:
  - Consider PCP if the patient is HIV-positive.
- If the patient has recently started ART, a worsening cough may be a sign of immune reconstitution syndrome (see 6.3).
- If the patient is taking d4T and has nausea or abdominal pain, consider lactic acidosis (a rare side-effect of d4T). Check the patient's lactate level.

Give supportive care:

- Give a beta-agonist inhaler for cough and wheezing.
- If the patient's shortness of breath is severe, consider a short course of prednisone 10-20 mg daily for seven days.

7.2 Hemoptysis

❖ Hemoptysis is dangerous if:

- There is a large amount of blood (patients die of asphyxiation, not blood loss), or if
- TB has not been treated.

❖ For large volume hemoptysis (> 200 cc, or a small cup), consider hospitalization. Call for advice.

❖ There is no good treatment for hemoptysis except for TB treatment. A cough suppressant such as codeine may decrease the frequency of episodes until TB treatment can be started.

❖ Hemoptysis may continue for months after the patient starts MDR-TB therapy. Chronic hemoptysis with small amounts of blood is not dangerous, and will resolve slowly as the lungs heals.

7.3 Persistent fever

❖ Fever due to TB may not improve for several months after a patient starts MDR-TB therapy.

❖ Consider the common causes of fever. See *Acute care*.

❖ If patient has recently started ART, new fevers may be a sign of immune reconstitution syndrome (see 6.3).

Give supportive care:

❖ Increase fluid intake. This is very important to prevent dehydration.

❖ Give paracetamol, but avoid an excessive dose. (see p.34.)

❖ The family may provide tepid sponging if the patient agrees.

7.4 Persistent nausea or vomiting

- Persistent nausea or vomiting is usually caused by ethionamide or PAS. Nausea due to AZT is usually of short duration.
  - Ethionamide has a direct toxic effect on the stomach lining and nausea is usually immediate.
  - PAS toxicity is usually more delayed.
- Both have a "dose-dependent" effect. Decreasing the dose will decrease the symptoms, which is why both are usually given in two daily doses.
- Decreasing the dose may increase the risk of treatment failure. Consult for advice.
- If a patient is taking d4T and is short of breath, consider lactic acidosis (a rare side-effect of d4T). Check their lactate level.

Give supportive care:

- Encourage the patient to continue treatment. Nausea and vomiting are often worse at the beginning of treatment when the body is very weak.
- Stagger the doses so patient does not have to take all drugs at once.
- The patient should take soft porridge before taking the doses.
- Increase the patient's fluid intake. This is very important to prevent dehydration. Offer the drinks the sick person likes, such as water, juice or tea. Ginger drinks can help. The patient should take the drinks slowly and frequently.
- Give metoclopramide (10 mg every eight hours, or 30-60 minutes before the doses).

7.5 Persistent diarrhoea

- Persistent diarrhoea may be caused by PAS.
- If the patient is HIV-positive, consider chronic infectious diarrhoea and treat it empirically.

Give supportive care:

- Increase the patient's fluid intake. This is very important to prevent dehydration. Give ORS if there is a large volume of diarrhoea. (See Fluid Plan B in ***Acute Care***).
- Give the patient a constipating drug unless there is blood in the stool or fever is present or if the patient is elderly, (see p.25 in *Palliative care.*)
- Advise on special care of the patient's rectal area, (see p.26 in *Palliative care.*)
- Advise on a supportive diet for patients with diarrhoea (see p.27 in *Palliative care*).

7.6 Peripheral neuropathy

- Many TB and HIV drugs can damage nerves and cause burning or tingling sensations. If the damage becomes permanent, these symptoms can continue even when the drug is stopped.
- If the patient is taking d4T, which is a common cause of neuropathy, switch to AZT.
- If cycloserine/terizidone or the injectable is causing neuropathy, discuss the risks and benefits of decreasing the dose or stopping these drugs. However, this may increase the risk of treatment failure. Consult for advice.

Give supportive care:

- Give the patient amitryptiline 25 mg at night. (If using carbamazepine, check LFTs.)
- Make sure the patient is taking pyridoxine.

7.7 Depression, anxiety or psychosis

- There are many causes of depression and anxiety in patients with MDR-TB, including socioeconomic problems.
- If the patient's symptoms are due to EFZ, consider switching to NVP.
- Severe depression, anxiety or psychosis is usually due to terizidone or cycloserine. Symptoms include:
  - Panic attacks
  - Hearing voices or seeing things that do not exist
  - Paranoia
  - Coma.
- Symptoms usually improve when the dose of cycloserine is decreased. Stop cycloserine immediately if the patient is suicidal or psychotic.
- Decreasing the dose of cycloserine may increase the risk of treatment failure. Consult for advice.
- See *Acute care* for management of depression and anxiety.

7.8 Hypokalaemia (low potassium)

- Low potassium in a patient can be caused by vomiting, diarrhoea, drugs and other reasons. The symptoms can be puzzling and include any of the following: fatigue, cramps, numbness, paresthesias, leg weakness, palpitations, somnolence, and confusion. Low potassium is common in severely ill patients.
- The injectable drugs, particularly capreomycin, can cause hypokalaemia. It is a direct effect of the injectable on the kidneys (renal tubules), which start to excrete large amounts of electrolytes, the most important of which is potassium.
- It is important to check potassium on a regular basis whenever beginning to use an injectable, even if it is several months after starting a Category 4 regimen.
- Give the patient oral potassium and magnesium supplements, and check the potassium in a few days. In severe cases, intravenous replacement is needed. Call for advice.

7.9 Adverse effects of MDR-TB/ART co-treatment

Signs or symptoms	Response
Abdominal pain	May be caused by several drugs. The patient should take drugs with food (except for ddI or IDV). Treat symptomatically (see *Palliative care*)
Nausea, vomiting (see 7.4)	May be caused by many drugs. If due to ARV, they will often improve in a few weeks. If due to ethionamide or PAS, nausea or vomiting may be chronic. Check for other causes of vomiting (see *Acute care*) If mild, advise the patient to take drugs with porridge and treat symptomatically. If serious, rehydrate with ORS or IV line
Diarrhoea (see 7.5)	If due to ART, the diarrhoea will improve in a few weeks. If it is due to PAS, it may be chronic If the patient is dehydrated, re-hydrate with ORS or an IV line (see *Acute care*). Examine, and treat for other possible causes of diarrhoea
Fatigue	Consider hypokalaemia or renal failure as a cause. Check creatinine, potassium Consider anaemia as a cause and check haemoglobin. Consider hypothyroidism due to ethionamide and PAS and check TSH
Depression, anxiety, nightmares, psychosis (see 7.7)	These may be due to EFZ or cycloserine/terizidone. If they are due to EFZ, symptoms will usually last less than three weeks. Mild depression can be managed with amitryptiline at night (see *Acute care*). Call for advice or refer if the patient has severe depression or is suicidal or psychotic. Serious symptoms may improve with a decreased dose of cycloserine/terizidone
Itching of skin, skin rash	If these symptoms are mild, give an antihistamine and monitor closely. If the patient has recently started NVP and is not responding to antihistamine, consider changing NVP for EFZ If the itching is generalized, or there is skin peeling, mucosal involvement, or other symptoms (fever, jaundice, etc.) stop all drugs (including CTX). This is very serious. Drugs will need to be reintroduced carefully when the rash has been resolved. Call for advice
Joint pains	Give non-steroidal anti-inflammatory (ibuprofen)

Signs or symptoms	**Response**
Jaundice (yellow skin or eyes)	Check the patient's liver function tests (AST, ALT, bilirubin) and stop all drugs. The jaundice may be due to EFZ, NVP, pyrazinamide or ethionamide or other drugs. Call for advice on how to restart drugs
Pallor: anaemia	Measure the patient's haemoglobin. Anaemia may be a sign of an undiagnosed OI. AZT may cause anaemia, often in the first four to six weeks. If the patient has severe pallor or very low haemoglobin (<8 g/dl; <7 g/dl in a pregnant woman), stop AZT/substitute d4T. Refer/consult
Neuropathy (burning sensation in feet)	This may be due to ddI, d4T, cycloserine/terizidone, isoniazid, injectable or other drugs. Stop stavudine and replace with zidovudine. If patient shows no improvement, start amitryptiline or carbamazepine (see *Acute care*) and call for advice
Muscle cramps, muscle spasms	The patient may have electrolyte wasting. Check potassium immediately; replace low potassium with bananas or potassium supplements
Headache	Give patient paracetamol. Assess for meningitis (see *Acute care*). If patient is on AZT or EFZ, reassure him/her that this is common and usually self-limited. If headaches are chronic, they may be due to cycloserine
Renal failure (swelling, decreased urine, hypertension)	Check creatinine. Stop injectable and call for advice
Hypothyroidism (fatigue, slowing)	Due to ethionamide and PAS. Do not stop any medications. Give thyroxine 50-100 mcg/day and recheck. The thyroid will return to normal once MDR-TB treatment is over
Fever	Check for common causes of fever (see *Acute care*). This could be a side-effect, an opportunistic infection or other new infection, or immune reconstitution syndrome. Call for advice or refer
Blue/black nails	Reassure. It is normal with AZT
Gradual hearing loss *(confirm that this is not due to ear wax)*	May be due to injectable. Refer or consult
Dizziness, lack of balance	May be due to injectable. Refer or consult
Changes in fat distribution	Due to d4T or ddI. Discuss this carefully with your patient—can she/he accept it?

8 Arrange follow-up and record data

Registration Group	Definition
1. New	Patients who have never received antituberculosis treatment, or who have received treatment for less than one month. This includes patients who had DST at the start of a Category 1 regimen and are then switched to a Category 4 regimen because of resistance
2. Relapse	Patients previously treated for tuberculosis who have been declared cured, and then are diagnosed with MDR-TB. This includes patients who had DST at the start of a Category 2 regimen and are then switched to a Category 4 regimen because of resistance
3. Treatment after default	Patients who return to treatment with confirmed MDR-TB after an interruption of treatment for two months or more. This includes patients who had DST at the start of a Category 2 regimen and are then switched to a Category 4 regimen because of resistance
4. Treatment after failure of Category 1	Patients who are started on a Category 4 regimen after the Category 1 regimen has failed
5. Treatment after failure of Category 2	Patients who are started on a Category 4 regimen after the Category 2 regimen has failed
6. Transfer in	Category 4 patients who have been transferred from another register for treatment of drug-resistant TB to continue Category 4 treatment. Their outcomes should be reported to the transferring unit so that it can report their outcomes in the cohort in which they originally started Category 4 treatment. This group is excluded from the quarterly reports of the receiving unit on registration and treatment when results are produced
7. Other	Category 4 patients who do not fit the above definition. This group includes Category 4 patients who were treated outside the Lesotho DOTS programme and for whom the outcome of the latest treatment is unknown

- ❖ Update the Category 4 Treatment Card. All data on the treatment supporter card and the facility-held card should be the same.
  - Weight: Write the patient's weight in the row that corresponds to the current month.
  - Observed doses: Copy exactly what the treatment supporter has marked in his/her treatment card since the last visit.
    - Morning dose: ⧄
    - Evening dose: ⧅
    - Both doses: ⊠
    - Refused to take drugs: ○
    - Self-administered therapy: →
  - New smear, culture data: Record any new smear or culture results on the treatment card.
  - Changes in treatment regimen: Record any change in treatment regimen, including changes in daily dosing.
- ❖ Follow-up form
  - Filled out by the doctor or nurse evaluating the patient at this visit.
  - Record symptoms and signs, adherence assessment and management plan.
  - Record the morning and evening doses of all medicines you are prescribing for the upcoming month.
  - Tick any side-effects in the box.
- ❖ If providing HIV care during the same visit, fill out the HIV Care/ART Card and file this with the Category 4 treatment card.
- ❖ File all lab results in the same folder as the treatment card.
- ❖ Dispense anti-TB drugs to the patient.
  - Explain the dosing of all drugs carefully, including ART and CTX, even if these are not dispensed at the same time.
- ❖ Schedule a follow-up appointment.
- ❖ Give lab slips for the follow-up appointment (see 3.3).
- ❖ Provide incentives and enablers to the patient and the treatment supporter.
  - Transportation support
  - Food package
  - Incentive for the treatment supporter.

Annex A: Education and support

A.1 Offer HIV counselling and testing

- All MDR-TB patients should be tested for HIV. If the patient's serostatus is not known, offer HIV testing as soon as possible.
- Pre-test information may be given by a physician, nurse or lay counsellor:

  1. Provide key information on HIV/AIDS.

  2. Explain procedures to safeguard confidentiality.

  3. Confirm willingness of patient to proceed with test and seek informed consent.

1. **Provide key information on HIV**

   Say: *"HIV is a virus or a germ that destroys the part of your body needed to defend a person from illness. The HIV test will determine whether you have been infected with the HIV virus. It is a simple blood test that will allow us to make a clearer diagnosis.*

   Following the test, we will be providing counselling services to talk more in-depth about HIV AIDS.

   If your test result is positive, we will provide you with information and services to manage your disease. This may include antiretroviral drugs and other medicines. In addition, we will help you with support for prevention and for disclosure.

   If it is negative, we will focus on ensuring you have access to services and commodities to help you remain negative."

2. Explain procedures to safeguard confidentiality

Say: *"The results of your HIV test will only be known to you and the medical team that will be treating you. This means the test results are confidential and it is against our facility's policy to share the results with anyone else without your permission. It is your decision to tell other people the results of this test."*

3. Confirm willingness of the patient to proceed with the test and seek informed consent

Informed consent means that the individual has been provided essential information about HIV/AIDS and HIV testing, has fully understood it, and based on this, has agreed to undergo an HIV test.

- "Unless you object, I will take a sample for HIV testing. I think it will be important for you to know this information. "

OR

- "I want to perform an HIV test today. If that is not all right, you need to let me know."

OR

- "I think this test will help me take care of your health and, unless you object, I'm going to obtain a sample. Can you agree with me?"
  If the patient has more questions, provide additional information. If the patient is unsure about or uncomfortable with proceeding with the HIV test or declines the test, make an appointment for a full pre-test counselling session. This session should address barriers to testing and re-offer the test.

If the patient is ready, then seek oral consent: *"In order to carry out this test, we need your consent."*

Remember: It is the patient's right to refuse an HIV test. HIV testing is **never mandatory**.

A.2 Post-test support

- ❖ Provide immediate support after the diagnosis.
- ❖ Provide emotional support.
- ❖ Provide time for the result to sink in.
- ❖ Empathize.
- ❖ Use good listening skills.
- ❖ Find out the immediate concerns of the patient and help:
  - Ask: what do you understand this result to mean? (Correct any misunderstandings of the disease).
  - Provide support.
  - What is the most important thing for you right now? Try to help address this need.
  - Tell them their feelings/reactions are valid and normal.
  - Mobilize resources to help them cope.
  - Help the patient solve pressing needs.
  - Talk about the immediate future—what are your plans for the next few days?
  - Advise how to deal with disclosure in the family. Stress importance of disclosure.
    - *Who do you think you can safely disclose the result to?*
    - *It is important to ensure that the people who know you are HIV infected can maintain confidentiality. Who needs to know? Who doesn't need to know?*
- ❖ Offer to involve a peer who is HIV-positive, has come to terms with his or her infection, and can provide help. (This is the patient's choice.)
- ❖ Advise the patient on how to involve their partner.
- ❖ Make sure the patient knows what psychological and practical social support services are available.
- ❖ Explain what treatment is available.
- ❖ Advise the patient on how to prevent spreading the infection.
- ❖ Ask the patient to return for a follow-up appointment depending on needs.

A.3 Prevent HIV transmission

- ❖ Warn the patient about the risks of unprotected sex and make an individual risk reduction plan.
- ❖ Educate the patient on the risk of passing their HIV infection to sexual partners.
- ❖ Facilitate HIV testing of partners (at a health facility or at home).
  - Explain that it is common for partners of PLHA to still be HIV negative.
  - HIV is not transmitted on every exposure.
  - HIV negative partners in discordant couples are at very high risk of infection.

A.4 Family planning

- ❖ Encourage condom use by all patients to protect from sexually transmitted infections (STIs), and to prevent transmission to sexual partners.
- ❖ Condoms are also an effective method of contraception when used correctly and consistently (offering dual protection from both pregnancy and STIs/HIV). However, if a woman desires additional pregnancy protection, she may wish to use condoms with another contraceptive method.
- ❖ Additional special considerations about contraception use for women with HIV include:
  - An intrauterine device (IUD) should not be inserted in a woman with gonorrhoea or chlamydia, or if a woman is at very high risk for these infections. Women with HIV or successfully treated AIDS can use the IUD.
  - If a woman is taking rifampicin, she should not use tablets, monthly injectables or implants as the contraceptive effectiveness may be lessened.
  - Spermicides, or barrier methods with spermicides, should not be used by women with HIV infection or AIDS.
  - Women on ART who are using hormonal methods are advised to also use condoms, as ART may reduce the contraceptive effectiveness.

Methods that are easy to provide				
Method	**How to use**	**Effectiveness (pregnancies per year in 100 women)**	**Common side-effects**	**Considerations for HIV-infected patients**
Male condom	Use every time you have sex	Highly effective when used correctly each time (two pregnancies per year). Less effective as commonly used (15 pregnancies per year)	No side-effects	Condoms are the only method that protects from STIs and the transmission of HIV
Female condon	Use every time you have sex	Effective when used correctly each time (five pregnancies per year). Less effective as commonly used (21 pregnancies per year)	No side-effects	Condoms are the only method that protects from STIs and transmission of HIV
Combined oral contraceptive pills or progesterone-only pills	Take a pill every day	Highly effective when used correctly (less than one pregnancy per year). Less effective as commonly used (eight pregnancies per year)	Menstrual changes, spotting, headaches, also possible nausea with combined pills	Women on ART should be advised to be very careful to take pills on time and consider using condoms for additional pregnancy protection and to avoid STIs and HIV transmission
Injectables (DMPA or NET-EN)	Get an injection every 3 months (DMPA) or 2 months (NET-EN)	Highly effective when used correctly (less than one pregnancy per year). Less effective as commonly used (three pregnancies per year)	Spotting at first, then no monthly bleeding; weight gain	Women on ART should be advised not to be late for injections

Referral methods	
Implant **Vasectomy** **Female sterilization** **IUD**	These methods provide long-term highly effective contraception and can be used by women with HIV

Emergency contraceptive pills	
	Provide to all women in case condom is not used, breaks or slips or as a back-up for other method

A.5 How to collect sputum samples

- ❖ A laboratory technician should stand behind the patient and supervise the sputum collection. Give the patient the labelled bottle, and bring him/her to the nearby open space far away from other people, and then instruct the patient by demonstrating with actual actions to:
  - Place both hands on the pelvis and either sit or squat.
  - Inhale deeply two to three times.
  - Open the container, bring it close to the mouth and bring the sputum out into it.
  - Do not give saliva or nasal secretions.
  - Close the bottle.
- ❖ Before the patient leaves the laboratory, visually examine the sputum sample for quality. If the sample is only saliva, ask the patient to cough again until a good quality sample is obtained.
- ❖ A good quality sample may require repetition of the procedure several times.
- ❖ Give the patient another bottle with the same laboratory serial number written on its side for an early morning specimen. Repeat the above instructions for bringing out sputum, adding that the patient should rinse his/her mouth with plain water before bringing up the early morning sputum specimen. This is to keep sample free of food particles. Food particles can appear like acid-fast bacilli under the microscope and can give a false-positive result.

Annex B: Care for health workers and lay providers

B.1 Personal protective equipment

- Regular face masks (that do not have a tight seal) do not protect against TB.
- Wear N95 masks over yournose and mouth when seeing any patient with suspected or confirmed TB. Make sure:
  - The nose clip is properly bent over the bridge of your nose.
  - Both elastic bands are in place.
  - There are no obvious gaps around the nose or cheeks.
- Check the fit of the N95 mask before entering a high risk area. Cover the filtration material with your hands and inhale. If there is a good face seal, it will suck up against your face.

B.2 Occupational health policy for health workers who have contact with TB patients

- ❖ This policy is applicable to any health worker who commonly encounters the patients with TB, not only those who work in the TB service, but also those who work with any patients who might have active TB (in outpatient clinics, inpatient wards, etc.).
- ❖ At baseline do:
  - A chest X-ray (if abnormal, it should be evaluated by a doctor);
  - A tuberculin skin test;
  - HIV testing and counselling strongly recommended;
- ❖ Annually: HIV testing and counselling strongly recommended;
- ❖ Any active health worker with cough > 2 weeks;
  - Do sputum smear microscropy, a sputum culture and DST, chest X-ray.

Statement on confidentiality

All health workers have the right to obtain medical treatment at any health facility, including the one where he/she works, without fear of disclosure of private medical information. Any health worker found to be discussing private medical information of a co-worker outside of a medical consultation with that co-worker will face penalties.

Acronyms

3TC	lamivudine
AIDS	Acquired Immunodeficiency Syndrome
ALT	Alanine Transaminase (a liver function test)
AST	Aspartate Transaminase (a liver function test)
ARV	antiretroviral
ART	antiretroviral therapy
AZT	azidothymidine—chemical name for the generic zidovudine
CBOs	community-based organizations
CD4	count of the lymphocytes with a CD4 surface marker per cubic millimetre of blood (mm^3)
Cfx	ciprofloxacin
Cm	capreomycin
cm	Centimetre
Cs	cycloserine
d4T	stavudine
ddI	didanosine
DST	drug susceptibility testing
E	ethambutol
EFZ	efavirenz
Eto	ethionamide
FBOs	faith-based organizations
H	isoniazid (INH)
HIV	Human Immunodeficiency Virus
IMAI	Integrated Management of Adolescent and Adult Illness
IMCI	Integrated Management of Childhood Illness
IMPAC	Integrated Management of Pregnancy and Childbirth
kg	kilogram
Km	kanamycin
Lfx	levofloxacin
Mfx	moxifloxacin
mg	milligram
NGOs	non-governmental organizations
NVP	nevirapine
OI	opportunistic infection
PMTCT	prevention of mother-to-child transmission (of HIV)
PAS	para-aminosalicylic acid
PEP	post-exposure prophylaxis
R	rifampicin
S	streptomycin
STI	sexually transmitted infection
TB	tuberculosis
Trd	terizidone
TSH	thyroid stimulating hormone
Z	pyrazinamide